Tumbling:

Learn to Flip, Not Flop

Authors

Cheryl Ann Hunter and Wendy Kay Bell

Copyright

Disclaimer:

This book is intended as an informational guide to the proper technique for conditioning, spotting and training involved in tumbling. The authors, Cheryl Ann Hunter and Wendy Kay, caution all readers to work with a professional who is certified in safety and coaching through a nationally recognized agency for gymnastics, tumbling and cheerleading. No one should attempt any of the tricks described in this book without a certified spotter and coach supervising the training. The authors do not condone "backyard training" and suggest that parents or team members who want to assist in spotting or training become certified in safety and coaching through a nationally recognized agency.

Table of Contents

Contents

Introduction

Cheerleading has become a major competitive sport in the past few decades. The level of skill, knowledge and talent necessary for successful and safe participation has reached an expectation of mastery that rivals Olympic gymnastics. This is especially true when it comes to tumbling skills. Much of the body conditioning for successful gymnastic skill is also necessary for cheer. Other activities such as acrobatic dance, urban gymnastics and sports such as skiing or skateboarding have also begun to tap into gymnastics. With the increased difficulty and physical demand of the skills and combinations comes added responsibility for both athlete and coach to focus on proper technique to help ensure safe execution.

Cheryl Hunter and Wendy Bell began coaching together in 1986 and have since put in thousands of hours of training and teaching to improve their knowledge. Cheryl started teaching tumbling for the youth for the city of Yucaipa during the summer of 1978. In 1979 she began working for a private gymnastics center in Redlands, and then moved on to help build a program for the YMCA in San Bernardino. Wendy began her gymnastics coaching career in 1986 when she was contracted to teach for the city of Fontana. She also assisted in teaching tumbling for the cheerleaders at Riverside Community College, where she later became a cheerleader herself. By 1986 the sister duo coached together at the YMCA until 1988 when Cheryl took a fulltime position elsewhere. In 1992 Cheryl and Wendy started their own program in their home town of Yucaipa, and later opened a full private competitive training gym.

Cheryl says, "As a competitive gymnast in my youth, and a coach and gym owner for over thirty years, I have had the opportunity to attend hundreds of hours of training from Olympic level coaches and physical fitness teachers to stay current on the latest methods of training. Athletic conditioning and proper preparation have always been the common theme. Without the proper conditioning an athlete (and coach) is put at greater risk of injury. During my years as a coach and gym owner, I maintained a safety and risk management professional coaching certification through USA Gymnastics.

Retired from the industry, I still have a love for the sport, which is why I have decided to share my years of experience to help athletes and their support system (parents, guardians, coaches, etc.) to be fully informed about how to safely learn their tricks and condition their body to increase longevity."

Wendy says, "My childhood was peppered with many sporting competitions, because I wanted to do everything. Baton, gymnastics, basketball, track, baseball, softball, and cheerleading gave me a well-rounded experience and knowledge of fitness. I have held certifications in USA Gymnastics as a skills evaluator, and professional certification in the disciplines of Women's, Men's, and Team Gym / Gymnastics. I also hold a certification in the National Academy of Sports Medicine. After retiring from gym ownership, I became a personal trainer.

I'm a firm believer in using your own body to reach tumbling goals with safe and achievable goals for those who do not have advanced equipment. My heart will always belong to the world of acrobatics, and my hope is to pass on my knowledge."

There are many different views about training techniques, but the experts are generally consistent in certain aspects. First is strength and flexibility preparation for proper execution of skills. Second is how to shape the body in the different phases of a trick in order to properly move through the motion and achieve the desired outcome. Third is the mental preparation that is necessary for an athlete to confidently follow through with the skill, avoiding injury due to "bailing out." Lastly, fourth is the importance of knowing how to fall properly, taking pain seriously and investigating any injury or strain that may lead to permanent damage.

Any professional, caring, and knowledgeable coach will emphasize these four points to maintain a safe and quality training program. Competitive sports for youth bring an obligation for adults to assure the health of the athlete. This is of utmost importance.

This book will take the reader from the basics through some advanced moves. There will be details on body positions, strength and flexibility and why they matter for each individual move. Suggestions on safe spotting will be included, with notes on danger zones to be aware of. By following the basic conditioning and preparation steps, most youth will learn the skills they need for basic cheer tumbling. Remember that everyone has a different combination of body type, strength, flexibility, spatial awareness, quickness and power, which means each youth will develop at different speeds. Patience and diligence are key. Rushing through the progression may lead to injury. Please be sure to read the author's disclaimer on the copyright page.

The reward of learning something new and achieving a goal is the satisfaction of accomplishment. Even the smallest improvement should be celebrated. Congratulations on your choice to improve your skills or learn something new, and best of luck to you in your acrobatic or cheerleading participation.

Section 1: Proper Preparation

Many youth entering the sport of cheerleading do so between the ages of eight and sixteen years old. These are crucial years for developing bone structure and major changes in body proportions. A youth may learn a skill before age ten and begin to struggle with skills at age twelve. Continual conditioning is important to help the youth adapt to the changes in body height, weight and proportion. This is not suggesting an increase in conditioning, simply a consistency. What was easy to do when a preteen, may become challenging after a growth spurt. Basics should be a consistent part of the weekly training to compensate gradually with changes in body proportions.

If a youth has never turned upside down, tried a straddle jump or put full body weight on their hands, there is the potential for injury. It is important to first condition their body and vestibular system to prepare for the new experience. Pay close attention to the wrists, since they may not have been conditioned for the amount of pressure that will be placed on them when executing a handstand, let alone a back handspring. Jumping and safe landing skills are important to ensure the athlete uses proper positioning of chest, knees and feet upon landing in order to avoid injury. Turning upside down and returning to a standing position without disorientation or dizziness is obviously necessary for safe skill execution. If a youth has never turned upside down, their vestibular (inner-ear balance) system may take some time to adjust to the movement.

This section provides preparation guidelines and suggestions for new tumblers however it may be a good refresher for those experienced athletes who may not have received such training before. The following will be covered: flexibility, strength, jumping and landing, wrist and ankle conditioning, safety falls, rolling.

Flexibility

Nearly every tumbling move requires some form of flexibility. Rolling forward or backward involves rounding the body into a tuck position with the neck bent and face into chest. Cartwheels demand some flexibility in the groin and hamstring. Back handsprings require stretching in the upper back and shoulders.

Before beginning any stretching activity, it is important to increase your blood flow and warm up the muscle tissue. This can be as simple as doing twenty five or so jumping jacks, running in place for a minute or two while doing boxing moves in the air, etc. Stretching may also be done following a cardio workout such as jogging, biking or swimming.

Activity to increase flexibility involves static stretching. The following are typical stretches used by gymnasts and tumblers.

1. Straddle sit

   The goal is to put your elbows on the ground in front of you.

   Begin by reaching over your right leg, stomach touching your thigh grabbing the foot with both hands. Hold the position without bouncing for a count of eight. Repeat on the left leg. Move your body to the center and hold for another count of eight trying to lower your body toward the ground in front. Be sure to keep the knees straight. Go through the pattern again three more times.

2. Lunge to split

   The goal is to eventually be able to split both legs, one in front and one behind sitting comfortably on the floor.

   Begin by stepping forward with your right leg and bending the front knee. Balance yourself with both hands on the ground. Position your foot so that you can see your toes when you look down, making sure your knee is right over the top of the foot, not in front of it. Keep your back leg as straight as possible as you lower your back knee on the ground with back foot facing down. Hold without bouncing for a count of eight. Repeat on the left leg.

3. Wrist and forearm

The goal is to loosen and flex the wrists and hands, as well as the forearms. Make a fist with both hands and roll them around making circles. Do this for a count of sixteen. Clasp hands together and rock them back and forth flexing one then the other eight times. Sit down on your knees and place your hands flat on the ground, fingers forward. Keeping your arms straight lean slightly forward to stretch the forearms and wrists. Hold for a count of eight. Stay on your knees and turn your hands around one at a time so that your fingers face backward. Hold for a count of eight.

4. Shoulders, neck and upper back

The goal is to loosen up your shoulders, neck and upper back. Sit in a cross-legged position. Put your arms behind your back and clasp your hands together. Sitting as tall as possible, turn your head to the right as far as you can and hold for a count of eight. Repeat turning to the left. With your head looking straight, bend your neck and press your chin to your chest. Hold for a count of eight. Slowly roll your head to the right, then slowly back to chest and then to the left. Roll your head back to center and slowly lift up. Slowly lift your head to look up as high as you can, then back to chest, then back to center. Staying as straight as possible, keeping hands clasped, try to raise the arms up behind you as high as possible, hold for a count of eight. Unclasp hands and lift them over head. Bend the left arm and grab the left elbow with your right hand, pull to the right over or behind your head. Hold for a count of eight. Repeat with the other arm.

5. Full back stretch *USE A SPOTTER UNTIL YOU ARE CONFIDENT

   The goal is to loosen and stretch your lower, mid and upper back. Stand with your back to a wall, feet shoulder's width apart and about two feet from the wall. Squeeze your buttocks and leg muscles allowing hips to move slightly forward. Lift your arms over your head and look up at your hands. Slowly reach back to touch the wall and then stand back straight. Repeat eight times. KEEP BUTTOCKS AND LEGS SQUEEZING THE ENTIRE TIME TO AVOID INJURY TO LOWER BACK. As this becomes easier, try it with your feet a little further from the wall. Within a few weeks you may be able to walk your hands down the wall and back up.

6. Bridge up from floor, tuck and roll (USE A SPOTTER AS NEEDED)

   The goal is to get a more complete stretch in your full back and learn to hold a comfortable bridge position. Lay flat on your back. Bend your knees and position your feet flat on the floor, heels against your buttocks. Bend your arms and place your hands flat on the floor under your shoulders, fingers pointing toward your back. Press with your arms and legs equally trying to push yourself off the ground. Keep your head neutral, not tucked and not too far back. Try to straighten your arms. Tuck your chin in, look at your stomach, then bend your arms and legs to slowly lower back to the ground. Bring your knees and chin to your chest, hold your knees with your hands and roll up then down, pressing your lower back out as you roll. Repeat the bridge, tuck and roll four times. BE SURE TO USE YOUR

BUTTOCKS, LEGS AND ARMS TO LIFT AND HOLD YOUR POSITION, NOT YOUR BACK.

7. Ankle conditioning

The goal is to loosen the ankles and work on their flexibility. Sit with your legs straight out in front. Cross one leg over the other and rotate the foot so that the ankle is slowly working. Do this for a count of eight, then switch to the other foot. Put legs straight out in front, tight together with knees facing up, muscles squeezing. Flex your feet as if you are pulling them back by the toes. You will feel it in the calf muscles if correct. Hold for a count of eight. Point your feet as if someone is forcing your toes to the floor in front of them. Hold for a count of eight. Repeat four times.

HELPFUL IMAGES

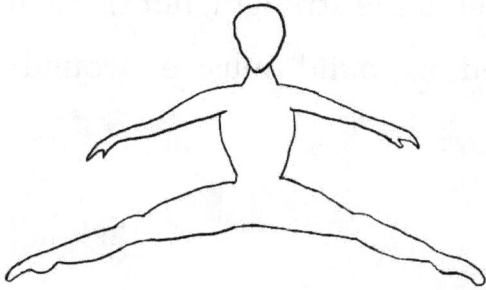

Straddle Sit

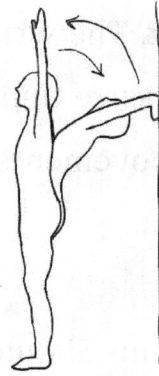

Back Wall Stretch

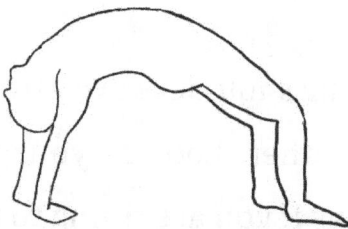

Bridge

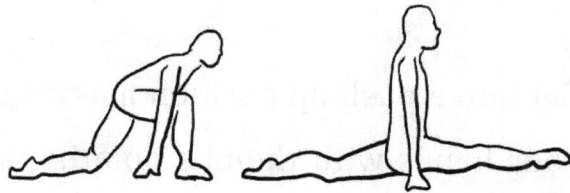

Lunge to Split

Strength

Gymnastics involves the entire physical system including spatial awareness, intuitive understanding of physics, strength, plyometrics, flexibility and focus. Strength is especially necessary in safely executing skills, but also to ensure good skeletal support. The wrists, elbows, knees, ankles, back and neck are areas of concern. Progressive tumbling helps to develop the strength, but there are also conditioning movements that are needed to build muscle around those vulnerable areas.

1. Wrists, Arms Shoulders

   The goal is to strengthen the wrists, arms and shoulders, but this activity will also strengthen the core (mid body areas). For those athletes who are still learning to do a safe handstand, this is a great progression or side station activity. The key is keeping the back straight, never arched during this exercise.

   Get into a push up position making sure your shoulders are directly over your hands with thumbs pointing at each other. Look at your toes and tighten your stomach and front of the body as if you are trying to pull your chest inward. Hold this position for a count of 30. Rest for a count of 30, then repeat the activity for another count of 30.

   Stand with your back to a bed, couch or mat stack, bend down to get into a push up position with your feet up on the surface, hands on the floor.

Follow step (a) again, this time pressing your shoulders to your ears. Make sure you are looking at your toes and tightening your stomach, bringing your chest inward.

From a standing position with feet together, bend down and touch the floor (do not lock the legs). Walk your hands out in front until you are in a full push up position, then walk your hands back, squat, then stand. Repeat ten times.

2. Stomach, Back and Hips

    The goal is to strengthen the stomach (lower and upper), back (especially lower) and hips (including buttocks and hip flexors). Nearly all tumbling skills involve the use of core areas and strengthening those areas will help to avoid injury, as well as improve the quality of the skill. For example, to execute a proper standing back tuck you must be able to lift your legs quickly toward your chest. This involves the hip flexor and stomach muscles. A back handspring requires strong back and buttocks to maintain the proper position during flight and snap down to landing.

    Lie face down on your stomach, legs together and arms straight out in front of you. While tightening your back and buttocks, and squeezing your legs together, lift your arms, head, chest and legs up off the floor. The only thing touching the floor should be your stomach and hips. Hold for a count of fifteen. Repeat five times.

Sit in a tuck position, arms stretched out in front, lift your feet off of the floor and hold the tuck position for a count of thirty. Repeat five times.

Lie on your back with your knees bent, legs slightly apart and feet flat on the floor. Lift the hips toward the ceiling by squeezing the buttocks and pressing down with the legs. Hold for a count of thirty. Repeat five times.

3. Legs, feet

The goal is to strengthen the legs, ankles and feet to prepare for jumping, running, leaping and landing. The more explosive the muscle can fire, the greater control you will have over quickness, rebound ability and height for executing tumbling skills. Plyometrics is a term for exercise that increases speed and power.

Stand with feet together. Bend your knees and jump to initiate movement, when feet return to ground rebound through ankles and feet ten times, trying to use only feet and ankles, keeping core and legs tight.

Stand with feet slightly apart, wider than hips. Bend your knees slightly and then straighten quickly into a jump while tightening your stomach, pressing through the feet and reaching your arms up. Upon landing, absorb by bending the knees and going right into the next jump. Complete three sets of ten jumps.

Stand with feet slightly apart, wider than hips. Bend the knees and jump as high as possible, bring knees to chest and back to landing as quick as possible, executing a tuck jump. Complete ten.

Stand with feet together, bend and jump as high as possible, straighten legs and move them apart into a straddle position, then back together before landing, bend the knees to absorb the landing. Complete ten.

4. Hollow body and back plank holds
   A "hollow body" is the term used to describe the inward pull of the chest and stomach forming a hollow or cupped shape to the front of the body. The muscles used to maintain this form are those used in many tumbling moves. It protects the back from arching during power moves and helps to hold the core with unified strength. One way to learn the hollow body is a back plank hold. Lie down on the floor on your back, place your heels on a stacked mat or other raised surface. Put arms over your head flat on the floor. Lift your body off the floor by tightening all the muscles and straightening the body like a plank of wood. If done correctly, the only part of the body touching a surface will be the heels and the upper back, head and arms.

HELPFUL IMAGES

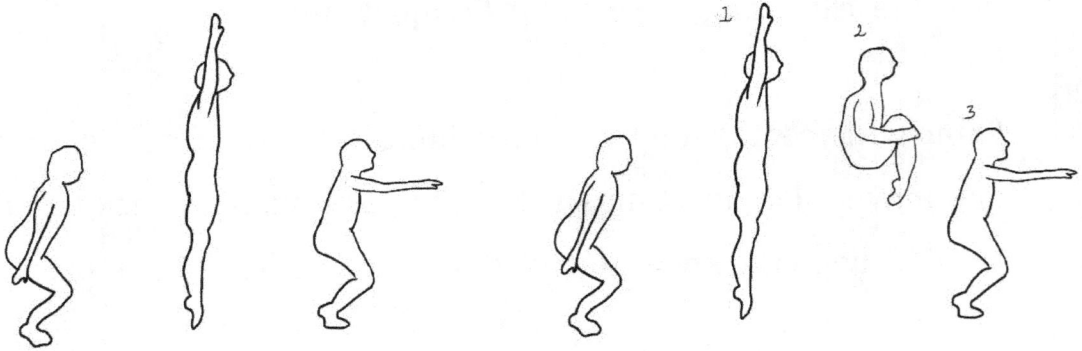

Straight Jump

Tuck Jump

Press through shoulders

Tighten and hold

Tighten and lift

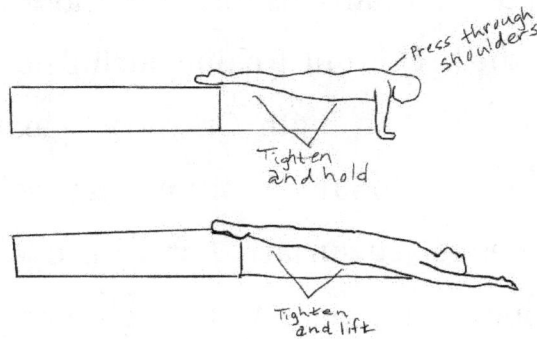

Front and Back Planks

Section 2: A rolling start

As we noted before, if an individual has never turned upside down or rolled forward, backward, it is important to orient the body to this movement prior to learning any more advanced tumbling skill. The following entry level tumbling skills should be mastered before moving to the next level.

Forward Roll

Begin by squatting with feet shoulder width apart, hands flat on the ground in front of knees. Lift the buttocks, slowly straightening the legs and leaning onto the hands. Tuck your nose toward your knees and lower the back of your head, upper back to the ground while bending arms. Let yourself slowly roll onto your upper back while maintaining a tight tuck position with chin to chest. Once this is mastered, begin to try adding the follow through to stand. In order to execute this without hands, the roll momentum should be continued by reaching forward after rolling, with feet pressing down and the body leaning into a squat to stand.

Spotting
Squat to the side of the tumbler with one hand gently holding their head in the tuck position while roll is initiated. Once the roll starts and the head is tucked properly, move both hands to the tumbler's hips and gently lift as the roll continues until the tumbler is safely rotated over onto their back.

Backward Roll

The backward roll is one of the most potentially dangerous skills to learn at the beginning level. Without proper assistance and technique, an individual may injure their back or neck. It is important to learn this skill for backward movement orientation development. A spotter is highly recommended. Begin in a squat position with knees against chest, chin tucked into chest and arms bent with hands at shoulders palms up. Maintaining this position throughout, roll backward and press the ground with hands as the back of head and shoulders contact the floor. Stay in the tuck position with eyes looking at knees and feet as the arms continue pushing to straighten as feet touch the floor. Press from squat to stand.

Spotting

Stand at the side of the tumbler with hands ready to grab the hips. As the tumbler rolls backward, grab the hips and slightly lift while the tumbler is rolling over to ensure there is less pressure on the head and neck.

Safety Rolls

One of the ways to reduce injury is to know how to fall safely. A safety roll is one that should become natural to all tumblers. Once the forward and backward roll has been mastered, the safety roll is easier to develop. The safety roll involves quick tucking and rolling with or without hands in order to protect the head and neck. The forward safety roll generally involves hands and arms only to momentarily guide the body--NOT TO STOP IT. The backward safety roll usually does not involve hands or arms as the goal is to prevent wrist and arm fractures when trying to stop a fall.

Good practice for safety rolls include:
Forward - learning dive rolls and front falling rolls.
Backward - learn to roll back from a standing position with arms overhead, pressing to stand

Dive Rolls or quick falling rolls

A dive roll sounds scary, and it can be. Start by learning a controlled pike roll (legs straight instead of tucked). Once that is comfortable, extend from squat to pike and immediately into the roll. Finally, put your arms up overhead, bend knees slightly, lean forward with hands aimed at ground, tuck your head and press your feet against the floor as legs straighten into a push landing on your hands and into a forward roll. Once this becomes comfortable, practice walking forward and just "falling" into a forward roll.

Spotting

The dive roll should never be attempted, even with a spotter, unless the tumbler has mastered the forward roll without spotting. Similar to forward roll, the spotter will stand to the side of the tumbler, but with hands on the tumbler's hips. As the tumbler begins to roll, hold the hips up slightly to keep weight off of the head in case the tumbler does not tuck properly.

Backward fall roll

To become comfortable with a backward safety fall, the tumbler should be able to squat and roll back without using their hands. Start from a standing position with arms overhead held tightly against the ears. Squat and roll backward keeping arms in the overhead position, body rounded and an open tuck with the legs. Once on your back, the rolling may be stopped by tightening the stomach and opening up the tuck. The goal is to roll back, but not to roll over. Eventually, this exercise may become a conditioning skill by adding a stand or a jump without using the hands and arms.

Spotting

The spotter simply needs to be ready to grab the hips to help the tumbler become more secure in rolling back without their hands. Also, initially help to slow the roll down at the end and make sure the arms remain overhead. Remind the tumbler to keep a tight stomach and open tuck to avoid knees hitting the face.

Backward straight arm rolls

The advantage of learning the straight arm backward roll is to practice keeping arms overhead when falling, and to know what to do if the roll momentum continues into a full roll. Keep the arms straight and press them back against the ground with the head tucked, then push to a stand once the legs come over.

Spotting

The spotter will grab the hips to lift gently in the same manner as spotting the backward roll.

HELPFUL IMAGES

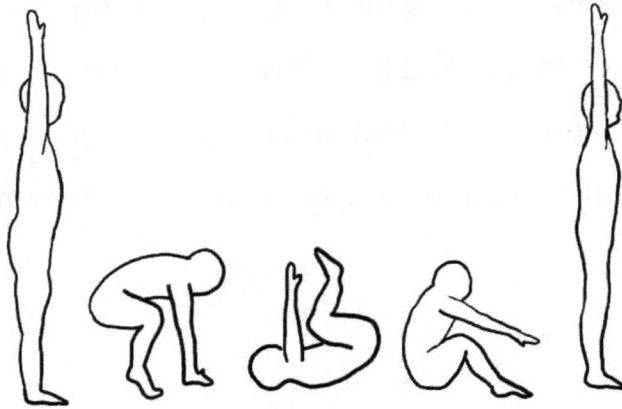

Forward Roll

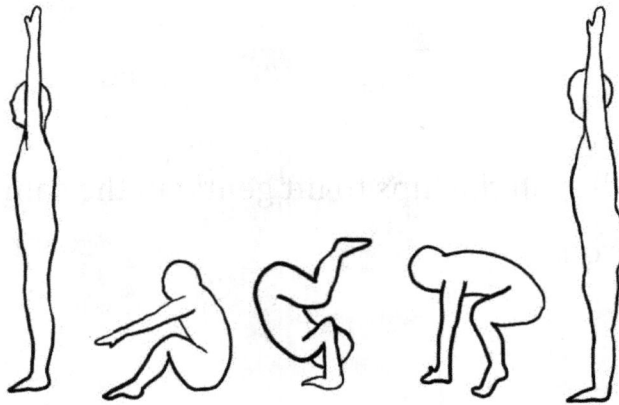

Backward Roll

Section 3: Handstands, Cartwheels and Roundoffs

With proper conditioning and having mastered forward, backward, and safety rolls, the next progression is inverted vertical skills.

Handstand

Executing a handstand safely and properly will lead to clean and successful cartwheels and roundoffs. The beginning drill to develop the proper handstand is an inverted lunge kick. With arms overhead pressed against ears, lunge with one leg forward knee bent and back leg straight behind. While trying to keep a straight line from fingertips to the toes of the straight back leg (like a teeter-totter), place your hands on the floor while lifting the back leg up. Keeping the back leg straight up behind you, with arms straight pressing against the floor, push off the other leg and try to bring it together with the leg that is up. Quickly bring the front leg back to its lunging position while still holding the back leg up. Repeat ten times.

Once this becomes more comfortable, the tumbler may try to get legs higher and higher. A handstand is not executed by kicking the back leg, rather it is done by a push off from the front leg and a lifting of the back leg. The proper angle of a handstand is with the head between the arms, chin neutral and eyes focused on hands. The stomach and buttocks should be tight with chest hollow (hollow body) and shoulders pressing to the ears. There should be no arch. Returning to the lunge should be a controlled movement maintaining the tightness of the entire body.

The spotter should stand to the side of the tumbler and grab the hips to ensure the tumbler does not fall forward on to head or land on the knees when coming back down.

Cartwheel

There are two basic types of cartwheels. One is with the body starting and ending facing the same direction throughout, just like a spoked wheel. The other is with a ¼ turn of the body going into and coming out of the skill. We will focus on the ¼ turn version, as that is what leads to learning the roundoff. It is important that the tumbler has already mastered the lunge kick before attempting the cartwheel, as it will develop their ability to hold the weight of their body on their hands.

Beginning cartwheels are much like beginning handstands, the body alignment should be straight from fingertips through toes of the back leg as if they are one piece. The difference is the ¼ turn of the body by reaching the second hand out in front of the first. Begin by lunging with arms against ears, body facing forward. The first hand will be the one on the same side of your body as the front lunging leg. Place the first hand on the ground in front of your foot as the back leg rises behind you. Reach the second hand out in front but in line with the first hand as you move the back leg over the top and press on the second hand. Your thumbs should point to each other. The foot in the air should land on the other side of the second hand. This sounds a bit complicated. But as shown in the image, an "around the corner" cartwheel is perfectly acceptable to start learning the motion. Remember that the cartwheel should end in the same position it started but facing the opposite direction. Keeping the arms against the ears is important to maintain the proper body shape as well as controlling the skill. The fully mastered cartwheel is one that begins in a standing lunge with arms overhead, is executed with as full a straddle as possible in the handstand position, then ending in the exact position as the start facing the opposite direction on a straight line.

Training tip: Place a small folded mat or cushion on the floor. Lunge into the cartwheel position with both arms against the ears and hands on the cushion. Try to kick the back leg around to land on the other side of the cushion.

Spotting

Much like the handstand, the spotter will assist by holding the hips of the tumbler. Stand behind the tumbler (on the side of the forward leg). Your hand that is the same side as the tumbler's front leg should reach to hold the hip of the back leg, while the other hand should be on the hip of the front leg. As the tumbler begins to move through the cartwheel, support the body by holding the hips and guiding them through to the landing on the other side.

Roundoff

The roundoff movements may be learned in a slow combination of body shapes prior to introducing the hurdle. It begins much like a cartwheel with a lunge facing forward, arms overhead tight against the ears. The first hand position placement is the same as the cartwheel. The second hand position placement will be reaching beyond the first, turned slightly in so that the thumb is pointing at you. The back leg will lift behind as with the cartwheel, and the lunging leg will push off, then meet the back leg to pass through the handstand, then the body turns as in the cartwheel but with legs together, feet landing at the same time.

The roundoff is a power move from the beginning. The back leg kicks forcefully behind as the front leg straightens quickly to press off the floor. The front leg should continue its forceful movement meeting the back leg through the top in a handstand position. At that point the movement continues with a forceful "snap down" of the body. The snap down is part of the success of a good roundoff. It is best practiced from a handstand position with feet against a wall or mat. It is properly executed with a slight pressing forward of the chest and upper arch in the shoulder area and a sudden return to the straight hollow position and a forceful snapping to the feet as the tumbler presses against the ground.

Once the snap down is mastered, and the roundoff basic movement is mastered. Practice trying to do the roundoff with the snap down from a lunge. When the tumbler can execute a strong roundoff without running, it is time to add the hurdle.

Tumbling Hurdle

The hurdle, or lag step, is a little skip between a quick run and the tumbling skill. The hurdle is done on the opposite leg of the front lunge. The tumbler must be able to skip first. Once the tumbler demonstrates the ability to skip, try to skip only on one side, as in step on one foot then hop on the other, then step then hop, etc. Repeat this drill on both sides. Using only the dominant side, practice stepping forward with one leg, hopping on it, then bring the other leg forward to lunge into a cartwheel. Make sure the arms are glued into the overhead position throughout the drill. This should not be done with a high kick, it is known as a lag step because the leg that swings forward to the lunge "lags" behind through the skip, then swings past the skipping leg and reaches forward into the lunge. There is no kick involved in the hurdle, it is the leg that hops that propels the body into the tumbling movement. Kicking causes the body to stop its forward motion.

Rebound

The rebound is a quick movement with the feet and ankles that is both the stopping of forward or backward motion and preparation for the next aerial trick in a sequence. When running and hurdling into a roundoff, the rebound transfers the snap down and traveling motion into a controlled vertical jump and safe landing to slow the momentum. Different from a jump from a squat, the rebound is a quick punch from the ground by pushing off the feet using the ankles and toes.

Run, hurdle, roundoff, rebound

Once the hurdle, roundoff, and rebound have been mastered, put them all together. Remember to lift your arms to your ears during the hurdle and keep them there all the way through each movement until the landing.

Training Tip: Be sure the "teeter-totter" alignment is maintained in the lunging position. The front foot needs to reach outward from the hurdle ready to push off. Equally important is hand placement. The first hand must be placed with the thumb facing in the traveling direction and the second arm should reach out as the legs join in the handstand position, and the hand should be placed with the fingers pointing toward the first hand (see image). This position allows the second arm to flex comfortably through the elbow and shoulder for added push off the ground.

HELPFUL IMAGES

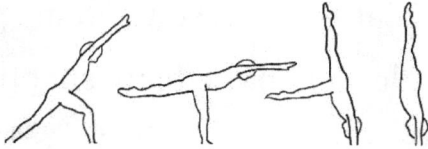

Handstand

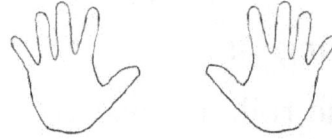

Hand Placement

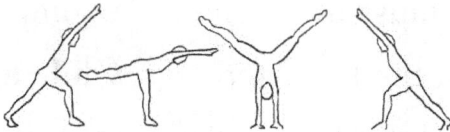

Cartwheel

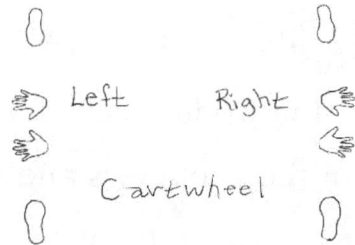

Hand Placement

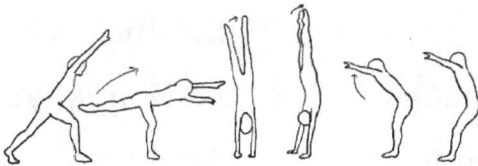

Roundoff

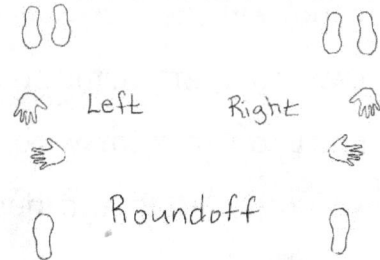

Hand Placement

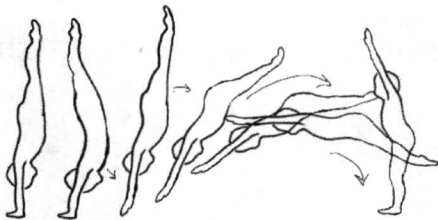

Snapdown

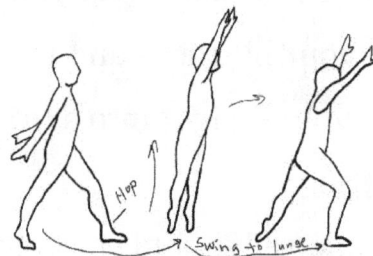

Hurdle

Section 4: Back handsprings

The number one goal of most tumblers is that second power move, the back handspring. Assuming the tumbler has already mastered a proper bridge, handstand and roll, the next step is to develop the basic body shaping drills to prepare for the back handspring.

Bridge back

First, the bridge back and kickover must be learned. This improves the flexibility in the shoulders and strength in the back and legs, while also going through the movements involved in a back handspring. The bridge back should always be done with a spotter in the beginning. Once it becomes comfortable with the spotter, then try walking down the wall or mat. Stand with feet shoulders width apart, arms stretched up against ears. Tighten buttocks and let the hips start to press forward as the weight shifts over the front of your feet. Look up at your hands and begin to reach further overhead, arms stretching through shoulders. Keep feet flat on the floor, allow the knees to bend slightly if necessary. As you reach over your head, notice that you can control your "fall" by tightening your buttocks and legs. Slowly allow your hands to touch the ground and center your weight into a bridge.

Spotting

The spotter should stand to the side of the tumbler with your outside arm reaching to hold the tumbler's opposite hip, and your inside arm supporting the upper back. As the tumbler begins to reach back, make sure the hips stay over the feet. DO NOT simply hold the lower back, make sure to support the upper back as the tumbler lowers into the bridge, this will support the lower back until the tumbler learns to use the proper muscles and body shaping.

Bridge kickover

The kickover is basically transferring the legs from one side of the body over the shoulders to the other side. The quickest way to learn is to push into a bridge with your feet on a mat or other surface that is at the height of your knees. Once in a solid bridge, rock slightly and lift one leg while pushing off the surface with the other. Split the legs, press down with your arms, shoulders to the ears and bring the front leg down, followed by the other landing in a lunge. When it becomes comfortable and easy, lower the surface until you are on the flat floor. Make sure that your buttocks and shoulders and stomach are squeezing and pressing, your lower back should not do anything other than bend.

Spotting

Stand to the side of the tumbler. Place one hand on the ribcage, the other on the lower back just above the tailbone of the tumbler. The object is to keep any pressure off of the lower back and make sure the tumbler does not collapse onto their head. Follow the kickover from beginning to end until tumbler is in the lunge position.

Back walkover, back limber

Once the bridge back and kickover have been mastered, try to put them together. With a spotter, stand with arms stretched up overhead, and the lifting leg straight out in front, toe lightly touching ground. Lift the front leg straight up and reach back into a bridge back allowing the kicking leg to continue moving over as arms reach back toward ground. When this becomes comfortable, try a back limber which involves both legs together pushing off the floor and lifting to handstand, then slowly down in front. ALWAYS USE A SPOTTER FOR THESE SKILLS.

Spotting

Stand on the dominant side of the tumbler and put your arm around the middle back area. Use the other hand to support the kicking leg. Follow the tumbler's movement as you support the back and assist with the leg lift. Be sure to keep the tumbler from collapsing onto their head and support the back by helping the tumbler to straighten through the handstand position.

Training Tip: Wall sits and Flybacks

The entry into a back handspring can be learned through a drill referred to as a flyback. It is a jump upward and backward onto a soft surface or into the arms of two spotters. Prior to learning the flyback, however, it is important to understand the proper body shaping for the first part of the back handspring. The proper take off position is with the knees slightly bent, over the heels and the hips bent as if sitting in a chair. To practice this position, sit against a wall.

The arms should be up against the ears. To do a flyback, jump up and back from this position landing in a straight tight body hold on a soft mat stack or into the arms of spotters. There is no need to swing the arms, as the force should come from the upper body as one unit combined with the force of the jump and straightening of the legs. Once the flyback is successfully mastered, it is time to follow through with the handstand and snap down.

Back handspring

Stand with feet together, arms stretched overhead against the ears. Bend the knees slightly and let hips sit back as you forcefully jump while reaching up and back into a handstand position, then snap down to a hollow stand, knees slightly bent through the landing. Be sure to squeeze the buttocks and stretch into an upper back shoulder arch as the hands contact the ground. DO NOT throw the head back, the arms should be against the ears and the eyes look for the ground, not the entire head.

Spotting

The spotter stands to the side of the tumbler with one arm on the center back and one arm under the thighs. If it is a small tumbler, the spotter may be able to be positioned on one knee. It is important that the spotter is in a position that allows them to hold the tumbler off the ground if something goes wrong. Two spotters is recommended unless the spotter is experienced. As the tumbler jumps the spotter follows the movement by supporting the back and helping to guide the legs. If all of the developmental drills have been accomplished and the tumbler is confident, this skill should be fairly simple to spot. If there are weaknesses and the spotter is having to do most of the work, then the tumbler needs more drills and development work.

HELPFUL IMAGES

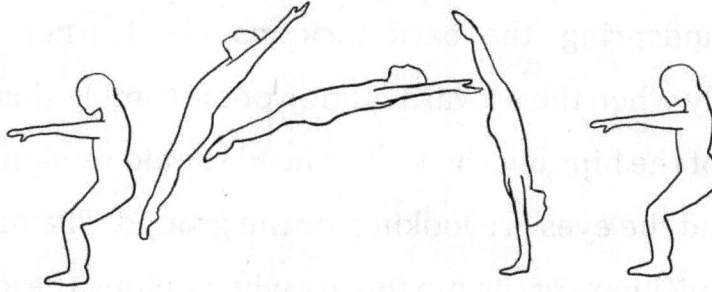

Standing back handspring

Section 5: Back Tuck (Salto)

The next back tumbling trick to master after the back handspring is the back tuck or salto. A standing back tuck needs quick-fire jumping and movement to be executed safely. Once a tumbler has mastered a proper tuck jump, basic rolls and back handspring, the back tuck may be learned. A back tuck is performed correctly when the upward motion of the tumbler becomes rotational due to the pulling of the hips overhead. The head should remain neutral until the body is inverted and the eyes are looking for the ground. The firing of the legs in the jump and the quickness of the hip flexors when pulling the knees and hips up are what create a successful back tuck.

Training Tip: Practice tuck jumps with a count of "1-2-3," where 1 is the jump, 2 is the tuck, 3 is the straightening to land. Count out loud through each position.

Tuck jump to mat stack drill

Begin with drills that involve jumping up into a tuck position and landing on a stack of mats or into two spotters' arms. Once able to land in a rolled back position, arms up and knees to your chest, move to the next step.

Standing back tuck

Stand on a firm stack of mats, about hip height, with a spotter next to you. Attempt the back tuck, with a spotter's help, by jumping up from the mat, swinging arms to your ears and bringing knees up to your chest, turning the tuck, looking for the floor, opening up for the landing.

Spotting

Stand to the side of the tumbler. Place your arm against the tumbler's back. Gently lift as the tumbler jumps and tucks, then use the other hand to make sure hips rise and turn over. Follow through with the tumbler by grabbing hips to make sure they land on their feet.

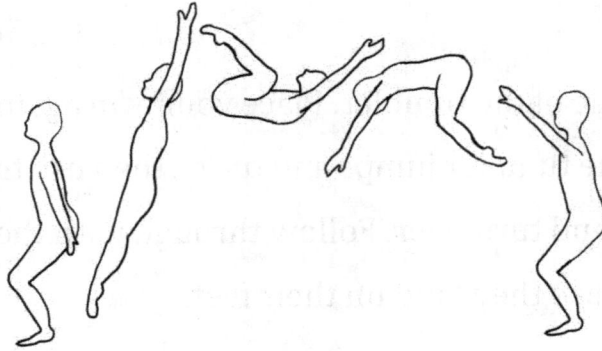

Standing Back Tuck

Section 6: Power Tumbling

This final section puts it all together with a basic tumbling run. The run, hurdle, roundoff, back handspring and back tuck is a basic competitive sequence of skills. The progression should begin with perfecting the hurdle to roundoff back handspring in order to develop proper body shaping and power from the snap down and rebound prior to adding the back tuck. When a tumbler can demonstrate a strong step hurdle roundoff back handspring to rebound, then they are ready to add the back tuck.

Snapdown to back handspring

Place hands on a stacked mat or firm surface (between 9 and 12 inches from floor). Kick to handstand and snapdown. While keeping eyes focused on the hands, follow through from snapdown to a back handspring and quick rebound. Arms should stay against ears throughout.

Spotting

Stand to the side of the tumbler, follow movement through the handstand and place your arm against the lower back as the tumbler's feet snap down to contact the floor. Provide support throughout the back handspring, ensuring safe landing and rebound.

Once the snapdown to back handspring rebound is consistent and comfortable, without a spotter, the tumbler is ready to take a short run and perform the roundoff back handspring. Spotting may be used for safety, but the tumbler should be able to complete the skill combination without lifting or heavy assistance from the spotter.

Run, hurdle, roundoff, back handspring, rebound

Take a few running steps, swing arms forward pressing the shoulders to the ears through a hurdle. Reach the lunging leg outward and execute a roundoff, shoulders to the ears throughout. Snap legs together quickly and snap down into the take off position, knees slightly bent, powerfully straighten legs and extend the body backward looking at the hands as they reach for the ground. Keep the arms pressing back, shoulders to ears with eyes looking for the floor. Upon contact, press through the arms and shoulders to perform a snapdown with quick rebound and safe landing.

<u>Spotting</u>

As stated before, spotting may be used for safety, but a tumbler should not be attempting the full combination until confident and ready, so there should not be a need for full assistance in the execution of the skills. The spotter should run alongside the tumbler and place hand under back as the back handspring is performed, just to ensure the follow through onto hands safely.

Adding the back tuck into the tumbling combination

The back tuck should not be attempted until the tumbler can show a properly executed standing back tuck. It must be demonstrated with arms in proper position and a control of the head (not throwing it back behind arms). The legs should extend fully through the jump with a quick pull to the tuck position and a controlled landing after rotation. Once the back tuck is mastered, and the roundoff back handspring rebound is mastered, the skills may be put together. The tuck is simply added to the rebound.

<u>Spotting</u>

The reason for spotting at this stage is safety in case of a bail out. If the tumbler tries to stop out of fear mid-air it may end in disaster. The spotter is there to ensure that the tumbler follows through and feels confident enough to complete the full series. The spotter should not be doing the work for the tumbler, but simply providing a supportive hand to ensure completion. Run alongside the tumbler, place hand on lower back through the back handspring and then follow the body movement through the rebound and support the back with a slight lift throughout the back tuck rotation. Place one hand on the stomach and one on the back to ensure a safe landing. As the tumbler becomes more confident, a slight touch of the lower back at the start of the rotation will be enough.

Closing Thoughts

A daily cardio workout is essential for sports such as gymnastics and cheerleading, as the continual movement and control of body shaping can be strenuous. Fatigue is a dangerous state for such athletes. Activities such as swimming, long distance running and aerobic dance workouts are simple options for building the endurance and breathing technique of an athlete.

Another beneficial practice is known as imagery. The visualization of a skill or set of skills, even a full routine has been proven to enhance the performance of the actual activity. It is a mental rehearsal of the action. The athlete imagines going through the skill or routine, attempting to fully physically "feel" the action. The most important aspect is in the perfect execution of the skill each time. Start with one skill at a time until the process becomes natural, then move on to a sequence and finally a full routine.

Video review is an excellent tool for perfecting a skill. The athlete can watch their technique, look for flaws in body positions, take off, etc. and then know where to make corrections. It is important to work with an experienced coach in this situation, however, because sometimes the adjustment may be as simple as poor hand placement. Young athletes may look at the aftereffect such as tumbling crooked and not realize it was the hand placement which started the problem. A good coach will be able to point out the steps in which the skill or sequence begin to fall apart.

We hope that this book has provided you with valuable information that may enhance and improve your tumbling ability. Dance and acrobatic movement are the oldest forms of physical expression. Gymnastics is the ultimate cross training activity. The level of achievement that the human athlete has reached is astounding, and we look forward to the new creative ways that future generations will take advantage of our ever-evolving physical ability as humans. Take pride in knowing that you are part of a unique club. We are so grateful to be a part of your success.

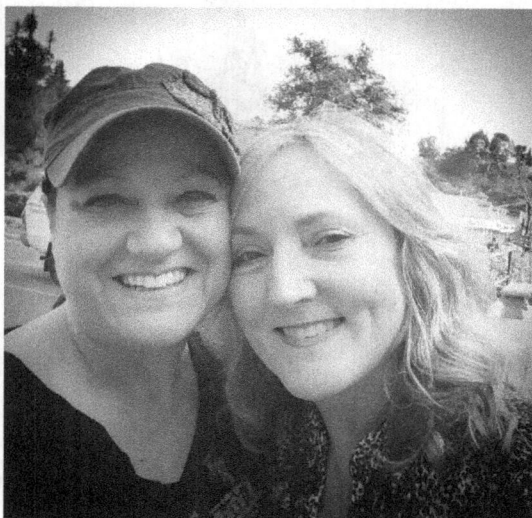

Cheryl Ann Hunter

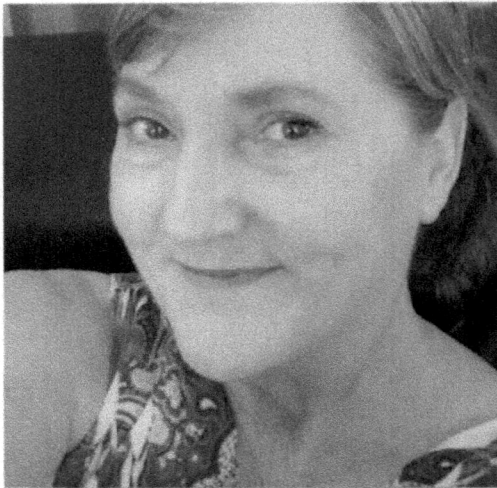

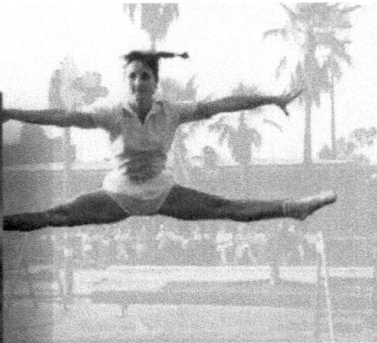

Cheryl is an author and artist living in southern California with her husband Mike. She has four children and three grandchildren.

Wendy Kay Bell

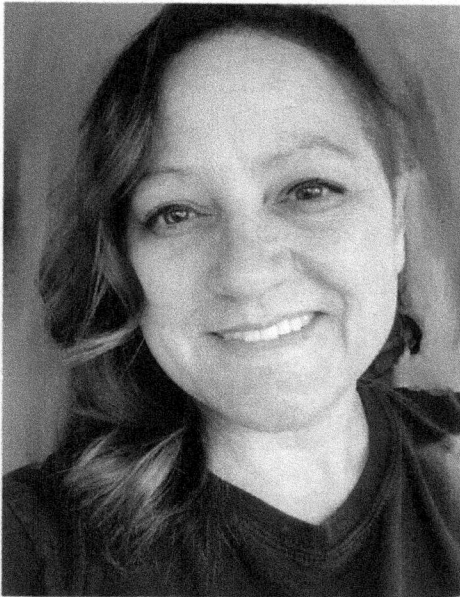

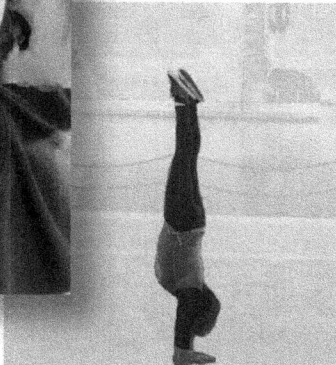

Wendy is a fitness trainer and
gardener living in southern California.
She has two children and one
grandchild.

Cheryl's timeline of experience:

1972 - Gymnastics lessons at Redlands YMCA

1976 to 1978 – Competitive gymnast for Yucaipa High School

1979 – Gymnastics teacher for city of Yucaipa

1980 – Gymnastics teacher for Redlands Gymnastics Center

1981 to 1990 – Gymnastics coach for San Bernardino YMCA

1987 to 1988 – Tumbling and Acro teacher for Redlands YMCA Circus

1990 to 1998 – Contract classes for city of Yucaipa with Wendy

1998 to 2012 – Co-Owner of private gymnastics training center with Wendy

2012 – Retired from coaching

Wendy's timeline of experience:

1975 - beginning level gymnastics lessons at Redlands gymnastics center.

1976 to 1978 - competitive gymnastics at Redlands Gymnastics center

1986 Coached for a recreation program in Riverside

1986 - Coach for YMCA San Bernardino

1987 to 1988 - Gymnastics Coach for Riverside community program

1988 - Coach for Carreras Gymnastics

1989 to 1990 Head Coach for San Bernardino YMCA gymnastics

1989 to 1991 Contractor for RCC summer gymnastics program

1992 to 1995 - Contract gymnastics for City of Fontana and Cypress Center

1992 to 1998 - Contract classes for City of Yucaipa with Cheryl

1998 to 2012 - Co-Owner of a private Gymnastics Training Center with Cheryl

2012 - 2016 Sole Proprietor of Tumble City

2019 - 2020 Personal fitness trainer

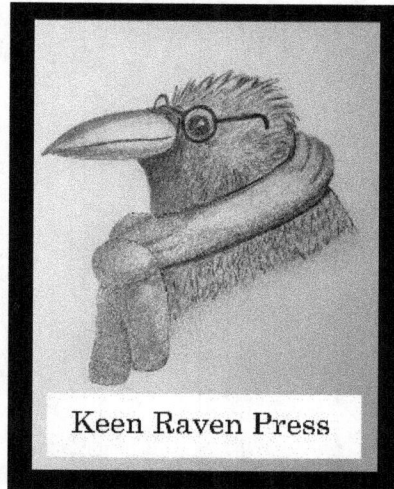

Keen Raven Press

Keen Raven Press is a southern California small publisher for independent authors. Publishing projects are selected based on the interest that the owner and managing editors have in the subject matter or any whimsical inspiration sparked by the submission. Email us at: info@keenravenpress.com

www.ingramcontent.com/pod-product-compliance
Lightning Source LLC
Chambersburg PA
CBHW081651270326
41933CB00018B/3433